A New Vibration

16 Simple Steps to Stay Lifted

Kiran Shashi

BALBOA.PRESS
A DIVISION OF HAY HOUSE

Balboa Press books may be ordered through booksellers or by contacting:

Balboa Press
A Division of Hay House
1663 Liberty Drive
Bloomington, IN 47403
www.balboapress.co.uk
1 (877) 407-4847

Because of the dynamic nature of the Internet, any web addresses or links contained in this book may have changed since publication and may no longer be valid. The views expressed in this work are solely those of the author and do not necessarily reflect the views of the publisher, and the publisher hereby disclaims any responsibility for them.

The author of this book does not dispense medical advice or prescribe the use of any technique as a form of treatment for physical, emotional, or medical problems without the advice of a physician, either directly or indirectly. The intent of the author is only to offer information of a general nature to help you in your quest for emotional and spiritual well-being. In the event you use any of the information in this book for yourself, which is your constitutional right, the author and the publisher assume no responsibility for your actions.

Any people depicted in stock imagery provided by Getty Images are models, and such images are being used for illustrative purposes only. Certain stock imagery © Getty Images.

Print information available on the last page.

ISBN: 978-1-9822-8158-8 (sc)
ISBN: 978-1-9822-8159-5 (e)

Balboa Press rev. date: 05/01/2020

Contents

Introduction vii

Part 1   Yoga 1

Part 2   Meditation 11

Part 3   Mindfulness 21

Part 4   Time 25

Part 5   Eating and Cooking 31

Part 6   Children and Animals 37

Part 7   Playing 43

Part 8   Clothes and Colours 47

Part 9   Your home and the places you go to 51

Part 10   Music and Dance 57

Part 11   People 61

Part 12   Nature 67

Part 13   Money 71

Part 14   Relationships 75

Part 15   Ego and Compassion 81

Part 16   The Self 85

Conclusion 89

About the Author 91

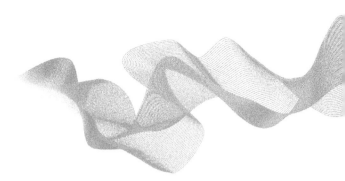

Introduction

Are there moments in your life when the more you strive, the less you seem to do, the more you search, the less you seem to find, and you suddenly realise that all the things you want you still don't have, and on top of all that you feel you're not who you truly are. If you have ever felt like that, then this book will show you a pathway to bring you more in touch with yourself and help you align onto your true-life path.

I know I have felt out of sorts sometimes. I clearly remember not so long ago at the age of 41 standing in my own presence with some fantastic experiences from my past and present, including the birth of my amazing son. I found myself saying, "I'm just not content. I want to attract my true vibrational life". I want to attract my vibrational tribe, my vibrational resources, my vibrational career, my vibrational location, and my vibrational love.' And then I took an in-depth look at my present life and asked myself, am I on that vibration anyway?' No, I am not. 'So how on earth can I attract that, when I am not on that Vibration yet?'

I questioned my self, my insecurity and security, my doubts and strengths, my view of love, how I nurture myself, how I give myself the time to 'just be' without judgements, and what resources I spent on my growth and healing.

In the months after that, I realised that even after 23 years of teaching Yoga, spirituality and wellbeing I still had to raise the vibrations in every part of my life if I wanted to change it. My outer life needed to mirror how I really felt and who I was on the inside. This book is the result of that journey, and I trust that it will help you too in your own quest for peace and contentment.

What lay behind that moment was the fact that I had separated from my partner three years previously. I was bringing up my lovely son without any support, and at the same time, I was running a successful well-being business, which was growing year by year. I was exhausted or, at least at times, I felt I was.

Every part of my life had been affecting me in some way. Whenever I felt 'I had things under control, and things made sense now', another part or subject of my existence would pull the rug from under my feet. In an instant, I would find myself back to feeling like I was at square one or at least faced with more feelings that I had managed to bury inside of me.

What I had to do was stop everything, step back and re-evaluate my whole being and my entire way of life by looking at each part of my life on its own and discover the many ways I could change the way I felt and what I reflected out into my world. It started with just watching my thoughts, positive and negative, and focusing on only those that empowered me. To replace negative thinking and to feel with a positive belief or affirmation is so incredibly hard, even for an experienced Yogi, especially when you honestly feel like rubbish! I watched how my emotions responded to my thoughts, which was usually a sudden pain in my middle back (on the right upper side to be specific) or pains in my neck. (Hence the famous saying) Eventually, i became aware of how I felt about those emotions consciously, which would then start to manifest in my physical body and my life as I knew it. Practicing Chakra work for me was a huge part of understanding the emotions and pains I carried within, recognising them, and letting them go.

I realised I needed to apply the same guiding principle to every part of my life, not just to some of it. I had to understand that my spirit, before I even became the walking, talking 'Kiran Shashi' here on earth had chosen to be here and to play its part, and it was up to me to enjoy it! Live it, breathe it, and embrace it fully! I realised acceptance and love for my self (and yes, Self-Love does not mean 'selfish, egotistical and egocentric. If you can't love yourself, how on earth do you expect anyone else too?!) was such a massive part of it!

I recognised that living life to its fullest comes with all kinds of emotions and feelings, obstacles and tests, pains, and celebrations. Still, the ability to bring mindfulness into my everyday life is one of the secrets to embracing it all. I also recognised the ability to practice meditation throughout my daily life, even in the awake state. Liberating myself from the illusions of the mind helped me to release the inner fight that was holding me back from feeling the peace and achieving my dreams. I realised I didn't have to be 'somewhere' or a label in society to be a success. I was already a success, and everything I needed to be by being alive, experiencing, teaching, giving, laughing, singing, dancing, eating, drinking, excepting, and not resisting. I was already everything that my son ever needed me to be.

Of course, living in this way is not always easy. Life throws things at us all the time. I am being tested continuously, and I am still learning. Occasionally life will surprise us with something that we could simply never comprehend or knew was coming, and we find ourselves yet again faced with another emotional test of inner strength. I remember one weekend I had just finished my workshop and left feeling so elated, but very soon after i was picking up my son and ended up in a horrible argument with my ex. At that time, I have to choose how to react and act. Do I operate from a place of fear and weakness or a position of trust, love, and strength? We could move from a moment of peace and joy to a moment of disagreement and being uncomfortable in an instant if we let our thoughts, emotions, and feelings get the better of us. One of those thoughts is, "how dare he/she mako mo fool, looo. I want to win this battle!" but, in truth, does it matter who wins the argument, or gets the last word in? Want we all want, is resolve, and to diffuse all animosity and be at peace. What will give you instant gratification in that one moment of winning may turn into a long-term guilt of making someone feel less or hurting someone. The "Warrior" is not Fear, anger, and hatred, but the opposite, a reflection of Peace, Love, and trust," The Warrior is the inner contentment of knowing who you are."

The truth is that everything will work out, just the way it should and always, for the good of the Universe. We just need to trust in that, and our life's journey becomes blissful and enjoyable. When we find ourselves in a situation where we need to dig deep, find that extra courage, and pull everything out of the bag, we always find a way to do it. We need to repeat to ourselves 'yes we can,' and 'yes we will! I have often found myself in situations that call for that extra courage, like finding myself with a very short window of time having to raise funds for something important or having to find the strength to create a whole workshop or seminar by a fixed deadline. I find myself digging deep within myself to solely provide the best for my son and yet still fulfil all of life's commitments by reminding myself that 'I am strength'. My affirmation at that time is "I have all the time I need" and giving myself a realistic action list to execute in the day (the important word there being 'realistic') including the action of 'play'. (Respect to the late Louise Hay, who's affirmation and mirror work have played such a positive role in my spiritual growth)

I think the fundamental thing I have learnt is that raising our vibrations is not something that we should do some of the time or only in some areas of our life, but all the time in every part of it. If I come out of a yoga class in bliss and then half an hour later, I am stressed and shouting about something; I am only dropping down to another level and back to the state of resistance and fear. That is why this book looks at raising the vibrations from different angles, in all parts of life. After all, we all live by our own perspectives in life and our own journeys. Realistically how can we judge another when we haven't seen what they have seen, felt, or ever walked in their shoes. Everyone's present emotions and feelings, including the decisions they take as a result of those feelings and emotions have originated from incidents in their current life and past lives. Everyone's version of life will reflect their own journey, learning, issues, and strengths. Some of us have acquired the spiritual wisdom at a very young age. It may be that their Karmic voyage brought them to this life on a higher vibration already, and it was just a matter of time before the realisation kicked in, and they remembered who they are. Once realisation happens, and the awakening occurs, we become part of the ripple that is continually growing bigger and bigger to create the gigantic wave of change that is coming for all of us!

So, as you might expect from a Yoga teacher there is a chapter on Yoga, mindfulness, and meditation as this will always be a strong foundation for me, my son, and our spiritual grounding, but my teaching and own learning has become so much more. Healing, spiritual growth, the awareness of our self and the planet can occur in so many ways, and this book is my way of igniting that spark that I trust will help anyone who reads it. In this book, I talk to you about the vibrational aspects of what we eat, the clothes we wear, the company we keep, the children and animals in our lives, and of course, our relationships with each other, ourselves, and to money. So often we compartmentalise these things and put them into separate realities, not realising that they are all inter-related. We often neglect some parts of our lives and, as a result, become unbalanced. We need to raise our vibrations in every aspect of our lives. So, please stay with me as I take you on this spiritually awakening journey.

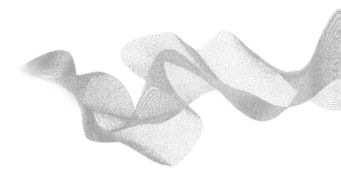

Part 1

Yoga

Yoga has been a part of my life for as long as I can remember. I started practising when I was at school. My family were all into holistic health and medicine. Some were yoga teachers or doctors specialising in Ayurvedic medicine, and my grandfather was a respected yogi. I don't remember him because he left home when I was very young, in search of further enlightenment, but my Mother often talks about him. I believe now as I follow his footsteps, he is constantly supporting and often amused, watching from the spirit world.

Yoga has always been in the family. I was practising it from such an early age that I didn't overthink it, I practised because it was just part of my life, and honestly, it made me feel good. I qualified in India during the last years of education and would often come back from school, sit down to meditate and do my Yoga practice as I felt it took me to another place of peace, and a connection to what I feel is 'home. I was that girl who would much rather meditate and perfect her headstands then spend hours on the phone to her friends chatting about things that honestly didn't matter. I understood the different dynamics between boys and girls quite early on and preferred to hang out with my big brother and his friends or just enjoy my own company.

Yoga and the spiritual way were always part of me. The practice of Yoga gives us so many things: more peace of mind, better health, it aids us if we want to practise meditation more deeply and of course, it raises our vibrations.

Yoga is more than physical postures

It is important to remember the true meaning of Yoga when we step into the practice of this magnificent art form that is the oldest recorded health system in the world. Yoga is the union of mind, body, and spirit. It is not just about the body. To practise the Yoga postures without mental discipline and without connecting to our spiritual essence would make it just a form of exercise. Which I would say is now quite apparent in the term 'Gym Yoga' or "become a Yoga teacher in a weekend."

Yoga has become so commercialised, in some ways egotistical, and is mostly promoted as a form of exercise. These days we have every Tom, Poonam, and Sally teaching and demonstrating Yoga postures, often converting it into a picture opportunity on social media or labeling themselves as a self-help guru by teaching or running seminars about an unconnected form of Yoga. I believe leading their followers entirely on the wrong path. When viewed and practised in this way, there is no connection to the spiritual consciousness, which is the main reason we do Yoga in the first place. It is taking the practitioner even further away from the spiritual awakening, enlightenment, and truth. These teachers, as I have said before, "The modern-day, quick Yoga Teachers," can be very Dangerous for the Universal good. The physical aspect of Yoga was created to strengthen and keep the body in good health, to be able to live a more present and embracing life, and also to sit through meditation. For someone unconnected to that and in dis-ease of mind and body would find it very difficult to get into the sitting postures to be able to meditate for long periods at a time. As you will see, if the body is experiencing physical pain, then the spirit is holding onto some emotional distress, which needs to be recognised, accepted, and released. For example, if you have pain in the joints, back, glutes, or the body is restless, you are certainly holding onto some emotional pain or trauma, which is mirroring itself to the outside world. The emotional pain could manifest in the form of someone or something that you consider a burden. Maybe you are taking on too much in your everyday life or perhaps, there is someone or something in your life that you see as "a pain.". All this emotional and physical pain makes meditation more difficult. The physical and mental discipline of Yoga is practiced to help you perform meditation and achieve spiritual enlightenment.

Don't strain, let go

When performing the Yoga asanas, we must let go of the desperate need to achieve the posture and release all resistance holding us back from achieving our highest state spiritually in the posture. Sometimes, we can get so caught up in the technique that we don't experience the liberation. The Yoga postures exist to guide us into the state of non – resistance, present state awareness, and being wholly at ease, no longer attached to the result and letting it be the decider of how we should feel. We must move away from the illusions of the mind, which act as the judge and jury, continually telling us how we think, how long we can hold a balance pose, or how far we can go into a stretch. We need to connect and become one with the posture and breathe into the posture. The more we become one with the asana and the act of performing the asana, instead of focusing on how we are delivering the asana and what we look like in it, the more we can let go of the outside worldly illusions distracting us from the present. We also need to pass through the mental and physical state of being uncomfortable in the posture, which leads to the resistance of performing the posture freely; this is done by accepting the feeling, embracing it, breathing through it, and releasing it.

Every posture that's practised needs to be in connection with the breath, which is the intermediary between the spiritual consciousness and the physical, this will lead to the connection with the higher vibration. The only way of doing a posture is by letting go of your three-dimensional being. What I mean by that is when you are physically doing a pose and pushing yourself to reach a desired point by forcing yourself to achieve it. It is much easier to let go and to let go of wanting to get to that desired point because when you surrender to the posture, the body relaxes, and you enter the space where there are no thoughts and then as if miraculously the position just happens.

If you just create the space and let go of your thoughts, you have then created the space to connect to the Higher Consciousness or Universal Intelligence, and that enables you to do the posture from the point of source. The space is also created to visualize yourself doing the pose. That is all you need to do: create the space and visualize yourself performing the posture. Visualization with an empty and focused mind is powerful and by clearing away the clutter from the mind, the Universe can intervene.

If someone is having difficulty doing this, I say to them: move away from your thoughts, take your thoughts back to the breath, to the oneness, a point of beauty, nature or focus on a point, or even a part of the body where you feel tension or pain. Focusing your attention on something present helps the person to enter the current state, and let go of the illusions filling up the mind. Then the spiritual connection can happen.

Towards wholeness

When connecting with the asana in mind, body, and spirit, we become one with our true selves. We connect with our identity and where we indeed are in our present state. Asana Yoga practised correctly is also a moving meditation. When we embrace our real state, the posture becomes true to us. When we let go of the restrictions and any inhibitors within ourselves, which I referred to earlier as the judge and jury creating the limitations, we can move with the practice more freely. An open mind can genuinely connect to the present and the higher vibration, we can then achieve more than we could ever comprehend. The Universe has suddenly taken over, and our mind has moved out of the way.

Understanding our real identity sits at the heart of Yoga. People often see their status as being a mother, a father, a wife, a husband, a singer, a painter, and more. The list could go on forever, but these are only labels that they have given to themselves. The tags are not really who they are. We are taught these labels from a very young age; education teaches us to be separate and not part of the whole. It continually teaches us to look ahead and not be present. What we are is an aspect of Spiritual Consciousness, the Universal Intelligence, the Spiritual Oneness experiencing itself through many forms. One of the purposes of Yoga is to make that connection with our spiritual consciousness, and when we make that connection, we understand who we truly are. It is finding the right path. We may work through 10 or 15 different careers in our lifetime, and then suddenly we see the career that truly resonates with us, in the 'now'. That is when we understand that our past working roles and jobs were leading us to this very point in time, to the end, when it becomes effortless.

Have you ever found yourself in that moment when you say to your self 'this feels right' 'everything just fits' 'like it was brought to me, even made for me'?

So, when we connect our mind, body, and spirit and let go of resistance, we can connect to our true self, which is the spiritual consciousness that is living through us, only then that consciousness can speak to us about who we are. You must be connected to your spiritual awareness to understand what your true identity is.

We often let the illusions of our mind and the ego override our spiritual understanding of infinite love. The ego becomes the reason we like to perform a posture. One of the reasons may be that we want to be recognised as the same as everybody else or better than others. We often feel the need to look our best and more to please others and this is very much driven these days by social media and the media on whole. This becomes the reason behind our act. When practising Yoga with that motive in mind, it will take us further away from the truth. We see so many people out there who base their worth on how many likes and followers they have on social media. It is so far away from the truth. They are more likely full of insecurities and need the constant massaging of the ego to keep them functioning in everyday life; they need the most help. A test for those people would be to cut away from the social media part of their life entirely for a while and see how their ego copes with no longer having the internet's approval.

Practising Yoga needs to come from the act of no resistance and the non-attachment to the ego so that the posture truly is about its connection to you and its benefit to you.

We achieve the deepest stretch not by pushing our body physically but by letting go of the desperation to achieve the deepest stretch. We accomplish the postures that once appeared to be so far out of reach by not trying too hard and straining to do them but by moving to the state of peace and ease and releasing resistance.

Try thinking of a Yoga posture that you practice that you would refer to as the hardest posture that you do or the posture that you hate. That is the posture for you to work with, to embrace and to get through because, at some point while performing that posture you will reach the point of resistance where it becomes uncomfortable for the body and mind, and you will reach your limit. At that point, it is crucial not to run away from that feeling and reach a block but instead, to get over it, to face it, accept it, embrace it and by bringing it into your present and move through your limits.

By connecting to how we feel inside while performing the posture and by recognising which tensions and pains show themselves to us, we relate to how we're feeling. Giving those tensions and anxieties our full attention and acknowledgment helps us to let them go. How can pain that is locked inside of us have the opportunity to heal if we don't recognise it? We need to let go of those trapped tensions and emotions by bringing them into the present state during our Yoga practice and letting them go with affection, attentiveness, and the breath.

It is important to recognise within your own self what your fears are and how they are affecting you living your life to the fullest. Remember that in real Yoga there are many branches to walk on. Hatha Yoga is only one part and, as I have already said, to practise the asanas without any connection and understanding of the mind, and the spiritual connection just makes it a physical exercise. It is not Yoga;

it is just a workout. Look at yourself in the mirror and your own life, and ask yourself, "Am I healed?" or "Am I at least in the process of healing"?

Teach when you are genuinely ready

There is absolutely no point in teaching Yoga when it is not from a position of truth, especially if you are only teaching for acknowledgment. What I mean is that teaching others when you are living in pain and unable to heal your self from mental and physical tensions due to the inability of being able to 'let go' is contradicting your teaching. You must learn to heal, love, and respect yourself first.

Becoming a yoga teacher or any spiritual teacher purely to feel accepted and feed your insecurities is not appropriate as it is an act led by the ego and not from the heart. The ego will always want acceptance and to be respected and looked upon with admiration. It wants to be loved and does it by creating fear within, fear of loss, fear of failure, fear of being alone, fear of not being respected, and more. Love exists inside of us not outside of us and that is the battle that we all have with the ego. Saying that, it is also important to remember that Ego is not the enemy. Ego is something we need in our life. It's the imbalance that is the problem.

We might begin our Yoga practice in a state of fear or anxiety and low vibrations, but if we just surrender and fully connect to our practice the truth will raise our vibrations to a higher wavelength. Connecting to our higher self and the infinite love is the goal. To teach it, first, you must become it!

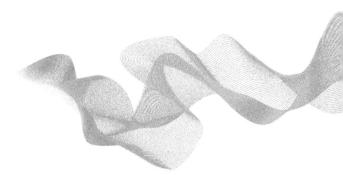

$\mathcal{P}art$ 2

$\mathcal{M}editation$

One of the things that has helped me most in my life is meditation. Meditation is not easy for all of us. Depending on our current life situation and our mind's preoccupation with past and future concerns, we can quickly become defeatists and give up on meditation due to lack of time, lack of energy, or even an inability to focus. It is difficult for the ego to understand why sitting and doing nothing could at all be helpful in the grand scheme of things.

When I first started doing more focused Meditation with my 6-year-old son, he would tell me how Meditation was "boring." He was already being conditioned by a system teaching him that he had to be busy and moving and that being still and creating space wasn't beneficial or fun. I found myself explaining to him that it was in the stillness and the space that great miracles would occur, it was in that state that control of the mind and body could be mastered.

I found Meditation helps me tremendously in my life. In the past, when I have found myself in situations where things were out of my control, and I didn't have any answers, simply being closer to the higher consciousness gave me peace and often the situation was resolved immediately. It was like my higher self or angels had intervened or by being in the state of peace, I had changed my vibrations to mirror who I was at that moment, creating a peaceful resolution to my problem. I remember a time, quite a while back now when I booked some flight tickets for my friend as she was traveling with us to the US for a family holiday, and somehow her name was spelt wrong on the ticket. I wasn't sure if it was my fault or the airlines, but when I called to see if the situation could be resolved, the airline said that a new ticket would have to be purchased for the total cost again. After going back and forth with the customer representative and then the manager, they said they would contact me back with the decision the following day and see if anything could be done but unlikely. I was agitated, and my friend couldn't afford another brand-new ticket at the time. This type of situation is easily resolved these days, but back then, it was more of an issue with some airlines. I didn't know what to do so that night I ended up meditating; I just let go for the feeling of peace to take over me. The following day when I spoke to the airline, the manager had decided it was a genuine mistake, and out of goodwill they would issue a new ticket at no extra cost. The relief was immense, but I remember thinking I had surrendered myself to the outcome as there was nothing more I could do and entered a state of peace and contentment. This practice also helped me through broken hearts. The practice of meditation is wonderful, because it enables you to be in the here and now and releases you from your worries and anxieties. There are different types of meditation practices, and each of us must find the technique that best suits us. Although I teach various exercises, I would never say that one meditation practice is better than the other. Different times in our lives call for different practices and techniques. Meditation is being in a constant state of present awareness and can be experienced in many ways. Sitting or being still in the present for long periods enables the meditator to quieten the mind and gain more clarity, peace, and a connection to the higher consciousness.

There are various meditation techniques, focusing on affirmations, a Sanskrit mantra, or on your breath, and there are meditation techniques where you simply listen or feel. Whichever method is used, meditation should lead to connecting with the Higher Consciousness, so you are letting go of all the illusions of your mind and merging with the 'all-knowing'. As you quieten the mind from thoughts of the past and future, you move away from physical attachments. It is bringing you fully into your present state of awareness.

You may need a reminder to bring you back to the present state, and therefore we say focus on your breath as your breath is the closest to the spiritual consciousness or focus on an element like fire or a candle, or even on a picture of your loved ones. Usually, when you look at these things, you tend to look at them from the outside only, you don't look at them from within. To be connected to the object of observation by also listening, feeling, and experiencing will silence the mind of other things.

I remember lying in bed one night, and my little boy was sleeping next to me. I must have just woken up out of a dream I was having, and I found myself tossing and turning. I tried to go back to sleep, but so many thoughts were racing in my mind, possibly triggered by the dream I just had. I then had a sudden thought, I couldn't hear my son. So, I slowly stopped thinking and listened. I listened for his breath, and there it was. Thus, warming, rhythmic, comforting, and quiet, and it just made me stop, or should I say made my thoughts just stop! I then felt it, the silence of the mind. It was so quiet with only the sound of my son's breath and absolutely no chatter from the mind. The peaceful feeling was an exhalation, a letting go, and it reminded me that this was the state I strive for during my Yoga and Meditation practice.

In meditation, you look at something from deep within going into its very core. When we bring someone's attention to the flame they can take the flame for granted, but when they really look at the flame looking deeper, they see the beautiful colours or the shapes that the flame is making and how it becomes bigger or smaller. We see the flame dancing. Suddenly, the flame has personality, character, and presence. The tiny flame suddenly shows huge 'Fire' potential. We need to appreciate the present.

Meditation is a beautiful, uplifting practice because when someone experiences meditation in its pure state, letting go of all illusions and letting go of perceptions about the past and the future and just listens, that feeling that you will have in meditation is euphoric. It is liberating. You suddenly connect to the highest consciousness of infinite love, and no words can give that feeling justice. It's almost like you've come home. The heart is lifted through meditation, leaving the practitioner with a much happier and lighter feeling. The bodies state is raised to a higher vibration. It is absolute bliss. And there is nothing hard about it, nothing that you must do. I never put pressure on myself to meditate.

If I go upstairs early in the day to meditate and my son wakes up early too, and he bounces upstairs and wants to play, then I go with that and practise present state mindfulness. And that is a form of meditation in its self. So, I'm entirely with him in the here and now that he is up. It would be completely pointless, me trying to fight that situation to find a quiet moment to sit and meditate. This is where I would need meditation to meet me instead of me meeting meditation. What I mean by that is meditation must fit into a person's life, not the other way around. Of course, sometimes I get irritated when I am unable to practice meditation as it has been said 'life gets in the way,' but then I catch myself, nip it in the bud quickly, and let the negative feelings pass. It has become easier to let go of things quickly over time due to practicing mediation techniques regularly, and this helps me to maintain a sense of inner calm when things around me are not. If you only meditate now and then it is not so easy to get out of a hectic state quickly. The more you practise meditation, it becomes a way of life, and the easier it becomes to maintain a quietness within, when your senses are assaulted by interruptions, the unexpected and the unwelcome.

You can also meditate just by going into nature, sitting by the sea, walking in the woods and listening to all the sounds around you and feel your connection to them. You will feel an instant lift, and that is one technique of meditation.

A busy life can get in the way, but...

Some people can meditate before their day starts, which is an ideal to aim for, However, for some, they'll find themselves in a slightly different situation. They wake up still tired from trying to get their child to sleep at night, and just about make it on time to take their child to school, or they can't find any time until they have finished their chores in the morning before they can sit down to do some quiet mediation.

Or for some, when they sit down to meditate, they are aware of the 100 or more things that pop up in their mind that need their attention, and the meditator literally cannot sit down for a peaceful 30 seconds. Sometimes you will find just as you sit down all enthusiastic about meditation; your eyes start to close, and sleep creeps in as you're so tired from everything you have done already in the day. It's important then, you do not force yourself but instead embrace your state and let go of the desperation to want to meditate.

In truth, the illusion of time can create the difficulty to sit and meditate, as we all run our lives by linear 'time' whether it be the number of hours we have in the day, or the amount of things we feel we should have achieved by a certain age. We can go deeper into 'time' later, but as quantum physicists have shown us for many years, the past, present, and future all exist at the same time. It is silly for us to put so much pressure on ourselves, letting linear time dictate to us.

A lot of the stress that people have today is because of financial worries. So, it does help to be more financially secure. It is also important to remember that wealth in its many forms is a vibrational energy itself, which we will talk about later, and which will attract its own vibration.

Dealing with financial worries is not easy. Often what is needed is reaching an acceptance of the situation. Once someone has entered the acceptance state, they will be able to find a way out. That is the process that they must go through, and it is not easy. One thing I say to people in that situation is to practise more present state awareness, be in the present more, and find more ways to enjoy the present moment. Find joy in every little thing that you possibly can, because that attitude will grow like a snowball and will manifest. It's sending a message to the Universe that you are grateful for everything that it is giving you so that the Universe will create space. The space will appear for things to manifest in your life that make it easier for you to meditate because your state has matched the vibration of mediation.

The person who doesn't have the money or doesn't have the time to meditate just needs to find joy in what they do have. You need to give up the fight, not give up on life, not give up on yourself and not give up on your children, just the battle. The battle is the problem because when you are fighting, you are in a state of resistance, you're not surrendering, not letting go. If the vibrational fight is always there, the Universe will give you the vibrational match. When you let go, a space is created within the mind's eye for messages to be sent down from the universe, which will give you the insight on which steps to take and which direction to move forwards on for your greater good. When you are grateful for what you have, the Universe gives you more.

Our whole day can be a kind of meditation

There is no right or wrong way to meditate. We can all change the way we feel about life by changing our thoughts, decisions, and choices, and the choices that we make give us all the time we need for our day. How we wake up in the morning, the first thoughts we have, and the first things we say to ourselves all have a positive or negative effect on our present state and then on how our day will run its course.

It may be that we just need to 'stop' for a minute and catch ourselves. Just listen to how we are feeling, what we are thinking, and watch what we are doing. Are we living in the present, or are we living in our thoughts? Just because we don't have the time to sit down and meditate doesn't mean we cannot meditate throughout our busy lives. Life itself can be one big constant walking meditation.

When we live life fully, and we are present in it, we can taste each part of it and savour the beautiful moments that we capture in our mind's eye. It is vital that when we see a beautiful moment, we don't just run to our camera to take a picture as we'll miss the feeling of the moment. We'll just be standing behind a lens and not giving ourselves the time to stand in the aura of the moment, embracing it fully with our complete self so that we can experience it in our mind's lens too.

The more we practise this, the more we enter, the higher vibrations throughout our day. The more things we can achieve throughout the day, the more energy we have, the better choices we make, and the quicker we make them. Life manifests the relaxed manifestation of being true to ourselves and letting it all go.

The Universe manifests what you are feeling. So, when you let go of your resistance, let go of the fight and let go of the illusions in your mind, you're fully in the present. You are then in a relaxed state of contentment, and that peaceful vibration will then manifest in your life.

Giving up your daily fears to the Universe and starting your day on the vibration of love brings people and situations in your life that mirror that state. We begin to find more and more time to do the things we most love, and those things continue to raise our vibrations. We even find the quiet time to sit down and meditate.

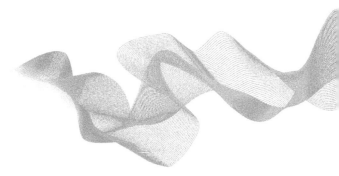

Part 3

Mindfulness

Mindfulness is being aware of our present state, and that includes not just ours but that of others too. Our location, the things we are holding onto, and with what mindset we go to bed at night all physically and internally affect our ability to be mindful. We find ourselves very thoughtful of our children and other loved ones in our lives, how they may be feeling or what they need etc, but can we practise the same mindfulness for ourselves and strangers?

Do we feed our body what it needs at the right times of the day, do we listen to our body if our internal organs are calling for rest, and a detox? Are we in tune and mindful of how our body is feeling when we are with certain people or discussing specific topics? Are we conscious of our planet, our surroundings, and other living souls?

Being mindful is being aware of our own emotions and feelings and accepting that others also have their own emotions and feelings, too, based on their perspectives, some of which we may not understand. When we take action are we reacting to a present situation, from past emotions or from fear of something in the future? Our own emotions and feelings about specific subjects or incidents or even how we feel about a person, in general, can influence our present actions and manifestations.

Can we watch the emotions that arise within us regularly as they can cause a knock-on effect in our present and future lives? Some of these emotions can push us off our path and ignite feelings that create anger, anxiety, or fear, which in turn manifest as tiredness, fatigue, and possible physical pain that can become acute or even chronic. Being mindful is distinguishing what's real from the fake and helps you to discern what is really behind your children's cries, your partner's outbursts, your own outbursts, the driver's road rage, and so on.

Mindfulness itself is also a moving meditation. It's being alive and present in all areas of your life, your home, relationships, your work, and when relaxing. To be able to change with all the circumstances that you find yourself in and to appreciate the beauty in all things is to become mindful. When being mindful, a person can see such beauty in moments of extreme sadness and vice versa.

Mindfulness is also about taking care of yourself, not in a selfish way, but acknowledging what your mind and body need. Are you mindful about what you eat and notice how some foods uplift you while others make you feel uncomfortable? I'm sure you've put something in your mouth, like a sugary donut or fried pakora, and thought it looked nice, tasted delicious, but after you find yourself not feeling too good. Are you mindful of the words and thoughts that you have and say about yourself? Catch your thoughts for a second when you are dressing up for a night out...is it, wow, I look amazing! Or well…that will do…. or uughhh I can't even look at myself? Are you saying good things to yourself during the day, or are you silently criticising yourself? It's important to catch your words throughout the day.

Saying negative things to yourself and others about yourself will only lower your vibrations. How many times in the day do you tell yourself and others 'I am tired'? At one point in my life, I found myself continually repeating that phrase every time anyone would ask how I was. It was after those words being my reply for a good year that I released 'no wonder I'm tired!' It's what I keep affirming about myself. My answer next time should be 'I'm great thanks' or 'doing good' 'really well' or whatever made me feel good. That vibration will manifest, and the Universe will find more ways to make me feel good instead of the old vibration of feeling tired. It is for the person to turn that negative into a positive. Positive words will raise the vibrations. You will feel better for it, and it will also make it easier for you to cope with the unexpected. The world around you will feel lighter.

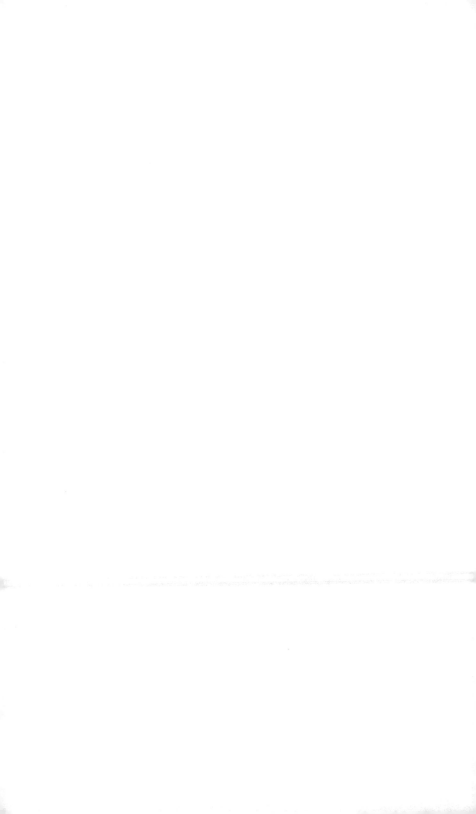

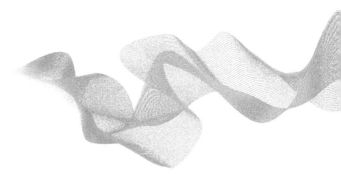

Part 4

Time

Are we slaves to time? Time within our 24-hour day or the pressures of time we put upon ourselves? Ironically this chapter on time was the last chapter I wrote while writing this book purely due to not having enough 'time'! I had to evaluate my own time Management.

Time really can dictate your every day, week, month, and year, but it is only when we become a slave to time that it becomes a matter of concern. When time seems to be going so quickly, and you find yourself chasing the clock throughout the day, it is then that we have a problem and need to 'stop' and look around us. With 101 things to complete and deadlines to meet we often put the pressure of timelines upon ourselves in order to stay in front of the crowd. These deadlines that we place upon ourselves are often part of our illusionary thinking that a project needs to be completed by a particular time, generally within the 24-hour day or within the 12-month year.

But when we look at it, why do deadlines even exist? Fair enough if you are working for somebody and they have given you a deadline, then you may need to complete a project within a time scale to present it to your employer. If you are sitting an exam or finishing some course work, you may need to finish by the given educational bodies deadline, but even those deadlines have been created by someone, for what reason? We just have to take their word for it. If you think about the school system alone, the ages the children start school vary. Some countries believe that children should start school at a young age as they can absorb things easier also they learn disciplines, formality and various subjects early on. Some countries believe children should start school later at the age of 6 when children have had the opportunity to 'just be' learned about the world from a far broader perspective. Some parents like to focus more on right-brain thinking, gaining, and learning the tools to live a life that is not of a controlled and regimented nature. Every deadline has been created by someone, often because someone before them has created the deadline and someone before them and so on. In fact, a deadline is often a pressure that we put upon ourselves. Living in a three-dimensional world, we feel controlled by what we call linear time and by our advancing age, so we put pressure on ourselves to reach certain milestones and achieve certain things by a particular time and by a certain age.

Some timings in our everyday life must be put in place, especially when there are trains to catch or planes to board. These schedules help the day-to-day running of the modern-day world. We may have a time slot on the radio or on digital TV to coincide with the school run or peak hour work traffic. We have appointments to make with various organisations because practitioners are only working or treating at a specific time in the day. But even a working day and time was set by somebody, and now more and more, every day we find that business owners are creating their own work timings. The once, 9 to 5 working day no longer suits or even is enough for most of the working population.

People also often live in fear of time as they put the pressure of time upon themselves. Looking at others in society, people often feel they need to achieve or acquire certain things by a certain age and put demands on themselves to get there within that time frame even if they are not practically or even emotionally ready. A great affirmation to repeat to yourself every day would be, "I have all the time I need" or "I am just where I supposed to be". It really helps to take the panic out a situation. People often find themselves depressed and suffering from anxiety because they haven't got what they thought they would have by a certain age. Yet, all these aesthetic or material things are an illusion. They are there and present if you are, and when the vibration changes, they can disappear or appear in an instant. Many people will stress they would like to be in a committed relationship by a certain age but for the ones that are, how quickly do we see divorces, separations or unhappy relationships, only for them to arrive back at square one, as far as time is concerned anyway. Similarly, we see people with blossoming businesses and everything they could dream of only to lose it due to some collapse in trading or because some family issue has intervened or a sudden twist in the stock market.

Everything is a vibration. It is not time that brings things to us but vibrational change. It is not time that takes something away from us but a vibrational shift. We don't bring things into our lives by chasing or pushing ourselves to get somewhere racing against time, but rather by entering a present state of awareness where time doesn't exist and where we mirror and manifest what we want to come to us. We can achieve the best health, wealth, success, family life, and more, but it can come to us at any time of our existence as those things will mirror our present inner state. The outer world is the reflection of our present vibrational state.

We have all the time we need really to reach those big goals because, to be honest, most of us do not know how much time - if we go by the invented 'age', 'year' and 'clock' - we have on this earth, so why are we rushing? It could be that we want to feel a certain way 'right now' and we believe that achieving or gaining something will help us feel that way. We pursue the object of our desire relentlessly as we firmly believe that once we have it, our goals are reached. This lifted feeling will last for a very short time until the next sense of wanting more appears, and again we put another timeline on ourselves for another objective, and we start all over again.

It is very healthy for the mind and body to step out of the restrictions and pressures of manmade time for a while, in order to give the person a chance to recuperate at their own pace. Holidays give us this, that's why it is so important to take those breaks away. It gives us more space to 'just be' and look at life from another perspective. It also helps our body adjust to other time zones and different ways of life, which then alter the stagnant vibrations within the body.

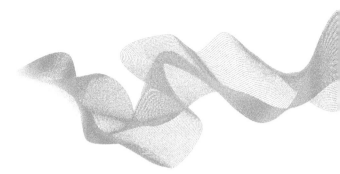

Part 5

Eating and Cooking

We are what we eat and what we eat we become. How can we expect to be on a healthy and vibrant wavelength if we consume things of a lower energy field? How can we expect to raise our vibrations when we eat and drink foods that have been changed, polluted or modified? How can we expect to raise ourselves to the vibration of love when we consume foods that are living in the vibration of fear?

It is becoming more and more important to look at how we are eating, what we are eating, how we cook food, and what oils we use etc. Are we eating organic or seasonal food, is it genetically modified, is it refined and processed, or is it natural? To eat foods that have been altered in some way cannot and will not be digested correctly within the body, and in retaliation, the body will send warning signals and react defensively as a resistance. To eat foods that were once part of a living, breathing soul is to consume all the feelings, hormones, and emotions of that animal. It is safe to say that no animal wants to go to slaughter and end up on somebody's plate for dinner to satisfy the consumer's taste buds.

A taste and greed that has manifested in an individual because of a disconnection with the living world. A suppression of compassion and a feeding of the ego will only lower the vibrations of the consumer and send out lower vibrational messages to their world.

Years of programming a child telling them that eating an animal's flesh is, in some way, good for them, along with the consumption of dairy foods, will make their taste buds and understanding know no better. So they will naturally develop an addiction to animal flesh and dairy. It will be challenging for them in their older years to eliminate those tastes from their diet. There is no end of delicious, nutritional, and healthy foods out there, and they are natural, plant-based, and uplifting.

Choosing the vegan route and way of life after being a meat eater and vegetarian for a big part of one's life can be very difficult. Foods never tried before or ingredients never used before in cooking and baking have become the norm. When a person first walks down the plant based path, it's an amazing realisation that animal products are 100% not needed in ay recipe. The concept that animal foods are necessary to us is something that may have been introduced to us at some point to satisfy the economy. Cakes and pastries, curries, and pizzas have been and can be made from 100% plant-based ingredients.

The body craves nutrients from foods that it has been aware of when growing up, generally before the age of seven, so it believes that the body can only obtain certain nutrients from those foods. I remember, through my pregnancy for a short time, I found myself craving chicken gravy, and I had to source plant-based produce to make up for the nutrients that I was craving, this was because I was brought up, in my early years as a meat-eater. Therefore, it is essential to bring up a child on the most nutritional foods that are not meat-based but plant-based from an early age. The adult moving forward from an awareness of compassion, intelligence, health, and a global awareness is the one that knows better. It is up to the adult to teach the child about being mindful of all living things and to explain that animals feel pain too, this should be done before dairy and meat become an addiction and a familiar taste in their everyday diet.

When eating a plant-based diet, the body and mind are lighter, calmer, and at peace, which helps lifts the vibrations to a higher wavelength. When eating meat and dairy, heat and anger is released in the body as well as toxins leading to a sluggish circulation. When we consume meat, we are imbibing the hormones and uric acids of the animal. Meat causes a lot of stress on the digestive system and produces heat within the body, creating a more irritable and angry temperament. Alkaline foods, on the other hand, create a cool sensation within the body. Alkaline foods are also easier to digest and take pressure off the bodies digestive system and well as calm the body.

The liver's reaction to dairy is to create mucus in the body to remove what it believes is a virus. That alone should make us think before we consume dairy. Lethargy can occur as a result of consuming dairy, osteoporosis has been noted as a symptom of diary too. Being tired and lethargic leads to a sluggish circulation which means that the body cannot flush out toxins.

Colds may also appear in the body, not to mention the many toxins that are released in the body from meat, chicken, fish, eggs, and dairy. More than three-quarters of the world's population cannot digest dairy, and that figure alone is something people need to think about before making dairy a huge part of their daily diet. I will not go into too much detail here regarding nutrition as I will discuss this subject in detail another time. Still, it is essential to realise the effect that food has upon us, not just physically but also mentally and spiritually.

Food has a 100% effect on our vibrations. So, if we want to raise our vibrations, we need to think about what we eat and drink. Do we want to consume food that drains us or food that makes us feel more alive and in tune with ourselves?

The Common perception is already changing

Raising a generation of children that do not understand the connection to other living souls and feel no compassion towards killing them in the most unimaginable ways only to consume them to satisfy the taste buds will manifest that negative reflection into society. A society of no compassion, love or understanding for others and a very violent world is born.

As people are becoming more aware of the health and worldly benefits of following a vegan diet, more tests and research is being done to ensure that the human being does receive all the essential nutrients needed to live with optimal nutrition as a part of their daily life.

It is important to question when watching and listening to other people's perspectives on this subject, even if they come from an educational background. The real question that should be asked to yourself is, "how do you feel?", not just physically as that will only be temporary but emotionally and spiritually about this?

The bigger picture and understanding are this, the outside world, including your body and internal organs, are a manifest of your thoughts and sense of reality. To be part of a world that consumes the vibration of 'fear' through meat and dairy will just help the vibration of 'fear' continue to manifest in your everyday life. You will always be looking for ways to feel better; any 'feel good' moment will be temporary. Only the fundamental change from 'fear' to 'Love' will ultimately manifest in a long-term healthy mind and body. If you feel you can't cut out meat and dairy entirely at least try to reduce it, the spirit and mind will respond, and eventually, you will feel a difference. It's important the change is not made through fear, self-righteousness, and dictating but through compassion, health, and the good of the universe.

Making the first conscious step forward will raise your vibrations, and you will mirror that out into your world, including your own body. The Universe will guide you into a healthier way of life.

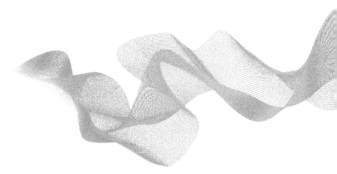

Part 6

Children and Animals

It's said that when you wish to become mindful and to be aware of your present simply spend more time with children and animals, as they are innocent images of God-consciousness and the closest to Source. Their innocence radiates unconditional, infinite love. They are natural in their ways. When my five-year-old son comes to my Wellbeing retreats, he is said to be one of the highlights, because he makes everyone feel better and lifts the group. If he thinks you look great in an outfit, he will tell you. If you come to the retreat feeling a little anxious, he is likely to say, "you look so lovely or you're awesome". He will spend time with you, talk to you, laugh with you and help you connect to your playful side. Children have no preconceptions, they don't judge, and they see the good in people.

Children bring us home to ourselves

Being around children and animals naturally brings us into a state of love and play where we have no choice but to let go of the illusions of our minds and just be. Their affection, their need for simplicity, and nothing more rubs off on us. Their appreciation of nature and beauty and the admiration of the little things in life helps us to connect to nature and raise our vibrations to the vibration of acceptance and love. Their enjoyment of the little things helps us to appreciate what we may take for granted.

Their mindfulness, when playing games or participating in an activity, shows us how to remain focused and be the greatest at what we also do. Their emotions are always real. If they're angry their angry, if they're scared, they're scared, if they're happy they're happy. Their honesty about what they see and feel teaches us to be true to ourselves and others and not to hold onto past and future emotional conflicts but let them be what they are in the present. So often we hide our true feelings about a person or situation for fear of not hurting others or not to rock the boat. Still, these fears will only hold us back from moving forwards in our life and may elongate a miserable situation even more.

Even when time spent with children and animals can seem tiring and exhausting, it still has a positive effect on your vibrations, as you're giving yourself wholly to them and having to be present. It is important to remember to stay lifted in that time. If you start becoming frustrated and the illusions of your mind get the better of you, the experience will become one of lowering your vibrations and an unpleasant experience for you and the children. You are giving yourself to their infinite love and respecting their innocence. You will see that they have no concept of time and rushing and being late, so it is very silly of us to keep repeating over and over that they need to hurry up. It is for us adults to work out how to get to where we want to go, and perhaps organise our time better.

Children are very much in the here and now and true to their own feelings and honest about what they see out there. If we are late, we feel the anxiousness, but they are 'just being,' and to them, it's difficult to understand the change in emotions of the adult. It is always important to remember that when hurrying the child or animal to get somewhere because they may have no concept of 'rushing', and the illusion of 'time'.

My son is constantly reminding me 'Mummy, there is no tomorrow' or 'there is no yesterday.'

It is also important when communicating with children or just being with children in general that your energy is as neutral as possible, so the child can be themselves and find their true selves. The situation may arise where the child completely imitates and takes on negative aspects of an adult only to become that vibration themselves. When they are older and have grown away from their childlike innocence, they will also start to manifest the negative traits of the adult. The adult can live by example for the children and walk and talk a positive way of life.

An animal also absorbs and feels the energy of the adult. When the adult is always angry or depressed or anxious, the animal or pet often takes on their owner's energy and will themselves start showing signs of depression, low energy and possibly become unwell. The animal is living an innocent energy in the present, which can be pulled one way or the other.

It is very difficult not to be in the present moment and connected to the higher vibration of infinite love when you are spending loving time with children and animals.

Laughing with children on our last retreat

Children can uplift us. On my previous retreat, we did a kid's yoga class, and it lightened up the group's energy tremendously. Everyone was invited to join in. The kids' class was practiced as a journey from the time they got up to the time they went to bed, and during that journey, they did many fun yoga postures.

Someone said it was one of the best classes they did, because everyone felt so free, and that's because kids don't think 'I must do the posture this way or that way', they just go ahead and do it, and If they fall over, they just pick themselves up and do it again. And believe it or not, they do the postures better than adults sometimes because they don't put pressure upon themselves; instead, they are so much more relaxed, and don't get embarrassed if they fall or find the posture difficult at the time. It's an experience for them, not a test or pressure they put upon themselves. They are so spontaneous and perform the Yoga posture to suit their own ability. There is no concern about having to look like everybody else. They have such a sense of fun.

Let growing Children 'be'

It's quite easy to feel that a child must be kept 'under control'. They live a significant part of their growing years in a formal educational system learning about 'being controlled' and learning about how to keep moving forwards because 'ahead' is apparently where all the rewards await.

I feel the educational system is to blame for categorizing children and trying to convince them of who they are and supposed to be. They are shown who is best among them and who is worst and where their place in the line should be. When I noticed this, and my son himself began to come home from school, explaining to me that one of his school friends were best at a particular subject. The other friend was best at another subject and he was 4th or 3rd best because that how it appeared to be, I decided to nip it in the bud quickly.

I explained to him that nobody was better than him, and to let anyone tell him where he should be in a line of best to worst is giving away his power. I explained to him to not wait for someone else to give him the 'best' accolade when they feel right but for him to 'take it' by aspiring, when he felt right.

I now see remarkable changes in everything he does after his belief changed.

We must show our children that life does have a structure, but that they can be free and flowing within that structure. For example, the soul in a singer comes from flow and freeness but they remain within the structure of a beat. They couldn't wholly be unconscious and unaware of this; otherwise, they wouldn't hear the beat and lose the rhythm. They would sound uneasy on the ear. The balance is so important to teach our children. That is the balance between the left and right brain. Our children teach us how to be free and flowing; let's not take that away from them for the need to 'control'.

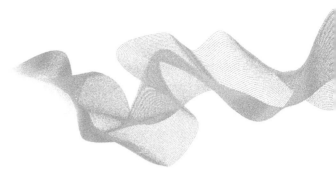

Part 7

Playing

Playing and being playful is one of the best ways to raise our vibrations. It truly lifts our energy, yet many of us fight shy of it. I think that when we grow up and become adults, we often feel that the playfulness must go, that life must be taken seriously. If we do play it may only be when we go on holiday, so that when we come back to 'real-life', we must be serious again.

There are so many benefits in allowing ourselves to play. When a person frees themselves of restraints like work and social deadlines, the to-do lists, action lists, work demands, and so on, the body and mind can be free, and it can let go. When the adult returns to the childlike carefree state that they once were their persona returns to the present and their vibration lifts to one of non-resistance.

Think about how you feel when you attend a comedy show, or sit back and watch a hilarious film, or have a whole day or night with friends and non-stop laughter. The following day will be a more relaxed, blessed, and lucky one as your vibrations will have been lifted through your own emotions and feelings. Your joy will have released any heaviness you had been carrying, which may have been creating feelings of fear within your mind and body, and you would find yourself in a place that is manifesting your higher state of consciousness.

That's why holidays are such a rejuvenating break as they clear our life of schedules, to-do lists, and timelines and let the individual 'just be'. I know there have been times when I have been away and left all my to-do lists behind until my return, only to gain more clients, more fun and surprises, and other opportunities upon my return.

Playfulness not only raises our vibrations of happiness, it also connects us more deeply to who we are. When you have fun and laugh, you return to the playful child within and return to your centre which is beneath and before the conditioning beliefs and destructive patterns that you may have acquired in everyday life. That brings us closer to the One Source that lies behind all creation. It feels as if we have come home. When we are connected to the higher Source, we are away from any negative thought patterns which can sabotage our free flow. These thoughts are very often other people's thoughts, other people perspectives, and opinions. When connected to the higher Consciousness, we are connected to our centre and we can create a space within us, away from past and future thoughts which are only the illusions of the mind then the right ideas and the right choices for our soul's life's calling can arise within us. Playfulness brings us back to ourselves and gives us a lightness of being.

From this playful, innocent centre where things do not need to be taken seriously all the time, everything in life can be appreciated. From this centre an understanding occurs that things just happen sometimes to all of us, and that we are not tied to anything that arises, we don't need to take everything to heart and so seriously. We begin to understand that it is just our emotions and feelings that arise from specific thoughts that fill our minds throughout the day, about the past and the future, and then the thoughts manifest in some form right before our eyes.

The illusions of the mind create a belief system within us, which causes us to take certain things so seriously to the point that they take over our day. If we moved forwards from a playful centre, we would probably laugh at the small things we at present consider a big deal and focus on the ones that are more important for our universal awareness and expansion.

Indeed, the feeling of laughter accompanied by the sense of letting go of resistance will raise your vibrations. If you take a few minutes a day to practice laughter 'Yoga,' you will feel lighter and less likely to take on negativity throughout the day.

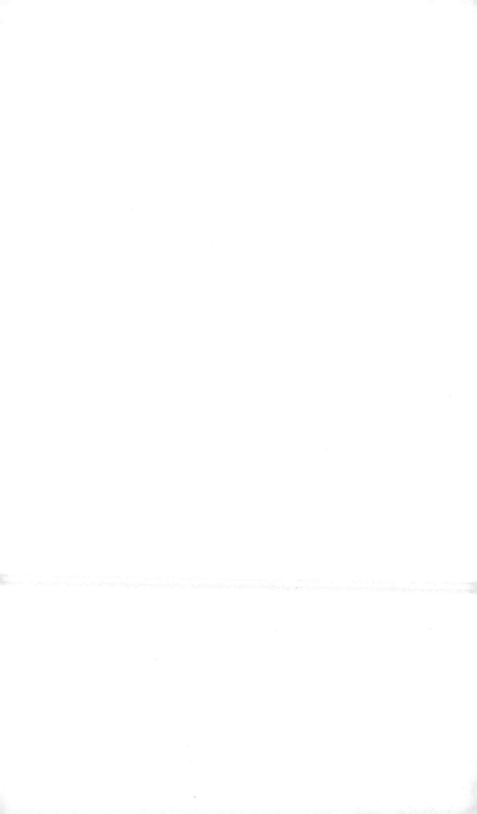

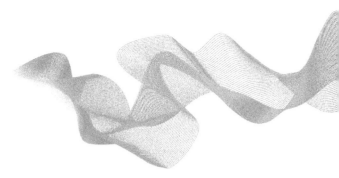

Part 8

Clothes and Colours

Clothes emit a strong vibration and can affect us more than we think. The clothes we wear can show the world what mood we're in and what we are in the process of doing. If we are casual or smartly dressed, if we have had time to get up and dress in the morning or if we have become overwhelmed with it all and dressing ourselves went right out of the window, it all shows itself in how we carry ourselves.

The colours we wear show us and the world how we are feeling. The colour of our clothes reflects if we feel confident today, or if we feel sexy, or if we want to be conservative, or be bold and make a statement or even discreet. It all creates an expression on our minds and energy, and on the other hand, if our clothes are very plain, old, and dull, again we often give off an energy that may appear less confident, shy, and we tend to step back from the attention of others.

It doesn't mean that a person must buy the most expensive clothing to resonate a positive vibration. A person that is dressed to suit their body and personality type will still resonate the higher vibration, and their confidence will shine. Whatever they wear, the belief system is essential here. What we genuinely believe becomes us, it will influence our vibration. So genuinely knowing that you can afford certain items, or that the Universe will move things in place so that you can afford to dress a certain way, will reflect in your energy field and you are more likely to manifest that which you desire.

Colours that we surround ourselves with, in our home, work, through the cars we drive, and, in the jewellery, we wear, all affect our vibration. Certain colours will also bring out specific energies from within the body, affecting our auric field and affecting the workings of our chakras.

Doing Chakra work with my clients, I have often found that my client will wear a colour subconsciously that matches the energy that they most desire and need in life.

Colours can also be attractive to energies from other dimensions, and some energies or even entities may find it easier to connect to us when we are wearing specific colours and are emitting a certain energy. The most significant way for any other outer energy to connect to you is through your vibration: the vibration of fear or love, and both Fear and Love can also be expressed with colours.

Wearing specific colours can lift our vibrations or lower them. When I run my weekend chakra course, I bring in a fashion designer, who works with everyone to help unblock any blocked chakras through colours and clothing. When you have a blocked chakra, the energy around that part of the body is constrained, causing emotional imbalance and sometimes resulting in a physical dis-ease, and the blockage will also manifest outward, holding you back in the reflective aspects of your life. The designer will suggest styles of clothing and particular colours that will free up and enhance a chakra. The result is that people feel happier, more confident, more expressive, and outgoing. It is incredible to see what a change in colours can do for someone's energy, and how that can raise their vibrations.

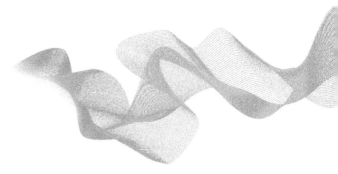

Part 9

Your home and the places you go to

The places we live in and go to are a huge representation of us and where we are, on our current spiritual journey. They influence our energy tremendously. They shape us in some way, and they can raise or lower our vibrations.

Living In an urban area surrounded by many buildings and people may have some benefits because you can create a family hive there and become part of a social circle. Still, that kind of environment can also be a source of low energy and spiritual imbalance that can affect you. For example, you are in an environment where you can easily be influenced by other people's thoughts and behaviours, especially if you are unable to have some quiet moments for yourself. Fresh air may not be easily accessible, and the closeness to nature may not exist in such a closed environment.

If you are living in a busy urban environment, it is so important to be able to create some space in your life where you can think your thoughts. Otherwise, it is so easy to feel bombarded continuously by what some people call 'the race of life' where everyone else's ideas and way of life become your own. It is also essential to take a little time out from family and friends and the people you communicate with every day just to be able to reflect and ground yourself in your being. It is essential to take a breath for yourself.

Being in a more suburban area surrounded by greenery, birds, animals, water, and space gives the spirit a chance to breathe and connect to its true self. In that kind of greener environment, you can feel closer to Nature and find it easier to enter the present state of awareness. Of course, living in such a situation can also have some low points, and someone may find themselves isolated and without connections. Loneliness can creep in, and that itself can lower a person's vibrations. If a person isn't of the mindset where they enjoy their own company and find love within themselves and what they do, they will need to be around other people to uplift them and give them love. So, balance is needed when deciding where to live, so where you live is in harmony with your spirit.

Take care of the vibrations of your home

Your home, however big or small, should represent you, your spirit, and your journey and be a clear and uplifting space for your soul to grow. The vibrations that enter your home are also important as your home is your foundation, so inviting someone of a scattered, heavy, fearful, or distorted vibration could change the energy of your home. The changes could affect you negatively, and you would feel them on an emotional and physical level. Also affecting the outer representations of the foundation energy field, your Root Chakra.

Keeping yourself clear, pure, and lifted is the first defence against other people's vibrations, as is also cleansing your home and surrounding yourself with positive words and quotes. Your uplifted spirit and vibration will itself become a defence for anything on a low wavelength. To keep yourself raised and in a positive state of love, keeps your frequency higher and you are much less likely to be attacked by a vibration coming from fear. An example would be something someone has said in conversation, an incident outside of you, or generally a cynical crowd. When your defences are down, and your energies are low, you can find yourself quickly in the vibration of fear, which will mirror and attract that lower vibration to you through people and situations also on a lower vibration. Similarly, that emotion may also arise in them when in your presence, as you could be on that vibration at times.

People can sometimes bring in a negative vibration quite unconsciously; they may be carrying anger or resentment about something that happened to them years and years ago. If you sense that someone has bought negative energy into your home, then after they have gone, you must cleanse your home. You should, in any case, cleanse your home regularly. That is not just good for you but also for your visitors.

So how should you cleanse your home? You can cleanse your home with the use of symbols such as Reiki symbols, or you can do it with crystals, candles, sage sticks, incense sticks, or with herbs or lemon and even affirmations. You will notice how much lighter your home feels afterward.

Locations around the world hold their energies and emotions. There are power points, or chakra points on Earth where energies accumulate, and these energies can be sent around the matrix grid that encircles the Earth to affect the world's entire population. An individual can harness these energies. When unsettling events are happening around the world, such as natural disasters, war, and famine, people of a higher and lighter power may decide to gather at specific high-powered energy centres and send out higher energies around the Earth's matrix grid. They can focus on sending their higher energies to the areas that need them most. They can send out peace and love to help others who may find themselves in a state of fear and suffering. Those people must be in a neutral state at the time and have love in their hearts for others. It would do more damage than good with people who generally do not like others as the ego and compassion would be imbalanced in that individual.

Holidays

The locations we choose to visit for holidays can sometimes call us and raise our vibrations when we most need it. It is essential to listen and be guided by your intuition and be led by love and not anxiety when making decisions about where to travel. I have met so many people who have been influenced by fear when planning their holidays. Fear of not having enough money, fear that their child might not travel well or become ill, fear that flights may be delayed, fear that they don't understand the location because it will be new to them or fear that they simply will not be safe. Fear that they will not be safe is a big issue for many people. However, a place that is regarded as unsafe might have a very high vibration. What is essential is to be in tune with your intuition and the higher consciousness, you will feel if your spirit feels safe and that can help you make a better decision for yourself.

If somebody in their heart wants to go to a new destination, the Universe wants them to go there for a reason. The money will be found, and it will work out, this always happens for me and friends of mine. If you trust instead of fear, the trust will take you where you need to be while Fear will stop you in your tracks. We continuously want to be in control, but the truth is we have absolutely no idea of the infinite possibilities that the Universe can bring to us.

When we feel lost or are struggling to find peace, and we travel to an uplifting location, our vibrations are raised, making a big difference to our lives. The energy of the place we are in, combined with the new-found peace and letting go of our everyday situation, will put us on a new wavelength. When that happens, it opens a door of new possibilities to enter our life, which matches our new lifted vibrations.

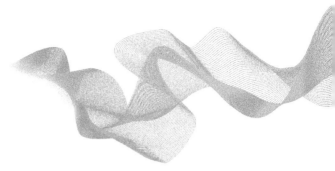

Part 10

Music and Dance

Music and dance are beautiful ways to lift our vibrations. Music lifts the heart and fills it with energy, and dancing releases the body's restrictions and tensions. Just listening to music can help us release trapped emotions that we may keep inside of us. The act of dancing is a 'letting go' and a creative expression of ourselves; it helps us recognise feelings that we are suppressing and uplifts us when we need it the most.

Different types of music can ignite various feelings and emotions and ultimately change our vibrations. Although all music has something in it to be appreciated, it is essential to think about how we want the music to make us feel. How do we want to feel throughout the day or how do we want to start and finish our day? For example, we may wish to hear uplifting music before a physical feat or competition, or we may wish to hear relaxing music with our child before they go off to school and so on. I often have some uplifting music playing in the background when I'm busy cooking in the kitchen.

Our vibrations can rise or fall with music, so it's essential to be aware of the style of music your listening too. A lot of commercial music is on a low vibration. Music that we hear on the radio is created according to a set format, and the notation of that format can often lower our vibration sometimes without us even knowing that it is doing so. We must listen as much as possible to music that raises our vibration and steer away from the lower forms. It is also significant to watch how you view and react to commercial artists. The Universal higher vibration does not idolise others; especially celebrity's out there, which may be on a very low vibration themselves. We need to protect ourselves from that anchor of fear.

Singing and playing instruments are lovely ways to express how we are feeling, and again a way to let go of situations and emotions that have manifested in and around us. To sing is to release the voice within that if kept inside can create anxiety and feelings of not being heard, which in turn would lower the body's vibration and could lead to a physical dis-ease like a sore throat, imbalanced thyroid and more. To sing is a way to express and speak up for ourselves when we feel we are not being heard. It is a passionate release.

Dance and let go!

I cannot praise dancing enough. Dancing releases the bodies pains and tensions developed over time from worries of the past or future. Dancing can help the individual to feel lighter and free and connect to their present. It is such a beautiful expression of the feminine energy of creativity and the life force and raises the body's vibrations to the higher vibration of love.

I often include dance in my wellbeing retreats, whether we bring in a Salsa teacher or convert one of our Yoga classes into play and dance.

Music and dancing connect people and bring them together. Everyone's energy is raised, and the vibrational high is lovely to experience. I've seen this many time. I remember being on holiday in Mexico some years ago, where there were two groups of holidaymakers staying in the same hotel. One evening lots of us found ourselves together in the same nightclub. There was dancing, and I was on the dance floor in minutes. Some people were quite happy to join, but the majority were reserved and sat and watched. I felt very; differently, I felt so free and completely let myself go, and because I was in that relaxed state I was able to get every single person in the group to dance with me one at a time.

One by one, they just let themselves go, and they became more and more confident in their dancing. Eventually, everyone was up on the dance floor, and I remember thinking to myself that some of these people had been very reserved and hadn't been talking to each other. Still, now they've come together in this experience and become part of the celebration of the evening - because everyone just let go. That's the power and the joy of music and dancing.

When you've been dancing, at the end of the evening, you're so free of physical tension and free of emotional stresses because dancing is such a liberation. You let go, your muscles are relaxed, and your vibrations are on a high. You are connected to the higher vibrations, and everything is connected, body, mind, and spirit. Dancing is an excellent tonic for the spirit. It's such a wonderful way to raise your vibrations.

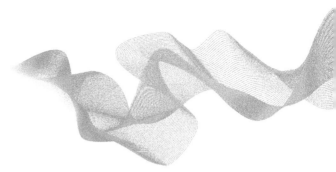

$\mathcal{P}art$ 11

$\mathcal{P}eople$

People do make the world go around. Meeting people, engaging, learning, helping, growing, and just hanging out with people can change your vibrations. People can raise your vibrations or lower them. People are walking talking masks living life, playing a part. Remember, every moment of every day it is just you and your thoughts, and if those thoughts become fearful or anxious in any way and you do not have the strength of mind to detach yourself from them and return to a positive vibration of trust and love then it's very likely you could quickly become your enemy.

Have an awareness of the vibrational level of what you hear

Your vibrations can change when other people are always in your space, especially when they are on a different wavelength and in a very different vibration. They could say something about a subject which can then become a thought in your head. That thought may then go around and round in your head with the result that you take yourself off a positive vibration that was manifesting good things for you and drop down to a lower vibration and start attracting something that you didn't want. That's why the people around us are significant. This can also be experienced in subliminal messages, which is more difficult to see. Just the awareness that subliminal messaging does exist will open you up to be aware of how you feel when you listen to music or see an advertising board; there may be a message in them to make you feel a certain way.

When someone says something to you, examine it, and if it doesn't feel right, counter it in your head with statements, you know to be true. For example, if like me, you believe that money is a strong and wholesome energy, and you hear someone say money is bad and causes problems, you can counteract that statement with positive affirmations in your head. You can say money is a blessing; it enables me to help people and animals and so on.

On the other hand, let's also remember that people can enhance and enlighten us and so raise our vibrations. Sometimes to bounce feelings, ideas, thoughts, and dreams off someone else gives you another perspective. That doesn't mean that you must listen to others all the time because everyone speaks from their perspective, but they may help you to make more sense of your feelings and thoughts and help you to see things more clearly for your benefit. While that can be very helpful, remember that people don't always give the best advice, because everyone is forever living from their vantage point, their journey, their past and future ideas. What is right for them could be bad for you, and what tastes good to them may not work well for you and vice versa

The joy of learning from others

We are all here to live our pathway, and that's the best bit about being here. Most of us find a niche in life and do what we are best at, and we realise that there are only so many things that we can physically do and know. But that is where the fun starts, because we are surrounded by so many people with different skills, different knowledge and different experiences whom we can teach us. We can learn so much from the path that others have walked upon. We can learn from those that have trod a path that we haven't or may have been afraid to walk on. Then there are others who went through some unimaginable feats for us all to benefit from the bigger picture.

The knowledge from the journeys that everyone has walked, and the wisdom learned from every individual soul will one day all return to the immense ocean of love for us all to tap into. Everyone's wisdom combined will help the spiritual consciousness grow and rise together.

It's also important that we are aware of other motives when learning. I often feel there are so many so-called 'gurus' out there spieling out what you should and shouldn't do. It's essential if you do listen, learn more from the one your heart jumps too as the heart feels the divine intelligence as opposed to making decisions from your head or stomach, which can be fear driven.

Connecting with ourselves and each other

Although people can sometimes be the reason for our pain and suffering, and we may feel that they lower our vibrations and make us feel defeated in some way, they can also help to lift us and act like our secret angels, coming to our aid when we need help the most. People can make us laugh when all we want to do is cry. They can help us see something that is right in front of us when we are just about to walk away from it. Something that we perceive as a negative act by somebody can turn out to be a positive act if we look at it from a bigger picture because, in the long run, it may push us to change something about our self that leads us to our soul purpose.

It's also true that some people work better together; hence we have our hive or our vibrational tribe, but everyone becomes our mirror at some point. Our own vibration attracts another vibration to us, and there is a connection, a mirror in there that brings the two people together for a reason. We invite to us a part of us that needs to learn and grow through another. It is because we are whole beings and we have a light and a dark side of our personality, and both sides need to be manifested. We are supposed to learn from our dark side, not be afraid of it. Some people enter our lives to rattle a fear we are deeply holding onto and struggling to let go. We may not feel these people are good for us at the time, but sometimes the ones that make us most uncomfortable are the ones that will help us to learn how to rise above the negative feelings that anchor us down.

Everybody has inside themselves a shadow side, something that they may not like about themselves, that they may not want to talk about and that they want to push away, but that very aspect of themselves can emerge in a situation and even create it. This can repeatedly happen, for example, in relationships. The reason is that the individuals in that relationship haven't looked at their shadow side. They may have been abused or bullied when they were younger, but they had never nurtured, healed, and dealt with that part of them. What they need to do is understand what happened and not hate it. It's about accepting what happened and not dismissing it.

We are all present and alive to help each other learn and grow, even if it is to realise what really does or doesn't fit us anymore. Deep down, we are all one and connected. We are spiritual beings living a human existence, and we do it through our perceptions, our viewpoint, and journey, the best way we know-how. We don't need to get on with everyone, but it is for us to respect others and their ideas and their journeys and let them be.

Are you with your right vibrational tribe?

What's important is having an awareness of what is your true vibrational tribe. This can change as we get older, and as our experiences and preferences change. So, at various stages of our life, we need to ask whether we are with the right tribe. Being in the right vibrational tribe will help us live our life's purpose and our soul's journey, but if we are mingling with the wrong people then we are most likely on the wrong track, and if things are not working out for us, we will probably know that we are with the wrong crowd. Once we realise that and change our path, maybe having moved into a different vibrational tribe, things will just flow more naturally. The Universe will bring to you the things that you need. The vibrational high of your tribe is essential to your life's flow, and it is so essential to create space between the people in your life who are bringing your vibrations down, because it is tough when you are with the wrong crowd to see where your path should be. So, think about the vibrational tribe that will best serve your life purpose.

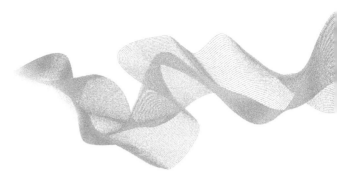

$\mathcal{P}art$ 12

$\mathcal{N}ature$

Our world and everything in it become us, in fact, it is us. We are connected to all and everything including the trees, the mountains, the oceans and skies, and even beyond the Earth we are connected to the planets, the solar system and the Universe. It is hard for us as physical beings living in this physical dimension to comprehend that we are a small part of the whole, and the whole exists in that small part. We are one little droplet in the entire ocean of life. We are all one, we are all entwined, and we are all connected to everything. We are all part of a higher vibration.

To think that of ourselves as separate from the whole is to reduce who we are. The knowledge that exists in another exists in you, and it is just a matter of connecting. We are one with the Universe so how can we hate any part of it, how can we hate any of our fellow brethren for they are also an expression of our selves. Even what we consider the most negative have somehow played their part in the bigger picture as without that act, certain acts of immense beauty may never have accrued. The Yin and Yang of life is always and must always be present.

Although we are all vibrating differently, we are all connected to the higher consciousness. Our vibrations will rise and lift once we realise and understand that. The Universal consciousness experiences itself through different forms, different dynamics, positives and negatives, different perceptions. This also makes it easier to understand multi-dimensional universes where the same individual could be having a completely different experience to themselves in another universe. If the Universe wants to experience everything, then we all must experience everything and every perception.

When everyday affairs consume us, and when we feel that it is more important to play a part in the so-called game of life, we can lose ourselves in the game, and then the game begins to pull us in. We start believing that everything in the game is real, that being in the game is who we truly are and that it is all there is, but when we do that, we cut ourselves off from the bigger picture. It is at times like that that we need to step back and remember that we are part of something so much bigger than ourselves. Nature can help us to do that.

Often when we can't find the peace within ourselves, we find ourselves admiring the beings who resonate peace and love. Standing in the natural majestic aura of a mountain and to 'just be', being strong and grounded, tall and fearless, or to stand with and embrace a tree and to root oneself into the Earth, into the here and now and stand tall connected to the sky is to be one with nature. Nature connects us with who we are. Nature is so close to the higher consciousness that when we connect with it, we see things differently. You can take the persona of parts of Nature to help you in your human journey. This is practiced through Yoga and Tai Chi.

To be one with Nature is to be balanced and flexible while remaining strong and standing. Sitting by the ocean is to remember that you are part of the ocean of love. Feel the waves of the ocean coming in and out and connect them with your own breath, your own inhalation and exhalation of life. Looking up at the sky and the huge, never-ending expanse of white and blue above us Is to let yourself go and immerse yourself in the beauty of the sky and the heavens.

When your spirit connects with Nature and floats into space, what its experiences is just pure, unconditional, infinite love. This can also happen when listening to birds, looking at flowers, watching blades of grass move in the wind, looking down dusty forest roads, and so much more. Nature, in its enormity, will bring you back into the present, the now and raise your vibrations to love.

Nature is also already within each of us. Its energy is present within us from birth. Many people often ignore this, because they have been conditioned and programmed into believing they must be a certain kind of person and behave in a certain way, but then sometimes their inner nature rebels because they realise that they have become something that they wish they were not. When that happens, Nature is erupting inside of us as it reacts with other elements of the outside world that no longer resonate with its wavelength. We need to connect our inner and outer nature to be on our spiritual path. When we are moving too far away from our true path, Nature will have a way of making us notice.

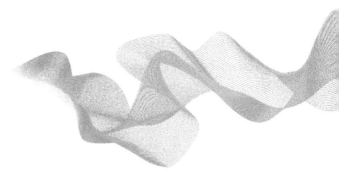

Part 13

Money

Money is another energy vibration. It has been said to be a lot of things: to some, it is the root of all evil, while for others it is a saviour or a means to help those living in difficult conditions. Money can be something that feeds the ego or something that can enable someone to flourish. Either way, is it the money or the way that it is used that is important? Money in its many forms can now be referred to as resources, notes, coins, chips, digits, cryptocurrency, and more. Is it an entity or an energy that rises and falls, that expands and contracts?

When we need it, can we call upon that energy, and when we don't need it, can we let that energy rest? The energy of 'getting and spending ', as William Wordsworth described it, can become a compulsion. That energy can consume us to the point where we see nothing else, and it becomes our primary drive to earn more and more to buy even more. It can engulf us and give birth to an ego that cannot live without the buzz of that energy, with the result that a person can lose their connection to their compassionate self. Once a person becomes ego-driven, the power of the money they acquire will match that and feed it.

On the other hand, can the energy of money feed compassion? It most certainly can. If you start from an energy of peace and love and a higher vibration, the money will grow to feed your compassion, and you will find money coming to you from every direction to help you. If you feel your life's mission is to spread an awareness of the higher self and others, then the Universe will provide the means to do this. Coming from a place of love, you will be working with the Universe helping people or maybe animals to lift their vibrations and help them live their lives as who they are. I've seen this happen.

I think a lot of people feel that to be spiritual, you must hate money and the making of money, and that is the problem. I don't agree with that at all. I believe you must love, embrace, and respect that vibration, because an energy will certainly not want to enter your energy field if you simply don't like it. If you are wanting to walk the spiritual path but understand you are very much 3-dimensional beings living in this 3-dimensional universe then money is a means to spread the spiritual awareness and knowledge; you want to have the means to help other people.

What is important is our relationship to money. Why is it when there is a financial crash some people are untouched by the effects of it? It is because their vibration and relationship to money is different from that of other people. For them, money is more than feeding the ego or satiating the fear of not having it; it is realising that help will always come and that they will always have all the money and resources that they need and more to do the things that they need to do. The money that comes to them is on a different vibration because *they* are on a different vibration. The energy that surrounds them is different from that of others.

It is important to look back to your childhood and be aware of where your money ideas have come from also to understand what your parents thought of money and how you saw money coming into your household. Was money hard to make back then, or did it come easily to you and your parents? This will often define how you see Money now and if your relationship with money is one of 'I have to work hard for money and to support my family' or 'Money comes easily to me, and I will always have all the money I need and more.'

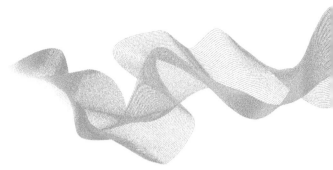

Part 14

Relationships

We have relationships of one kind or another in every part of our lives. They may be with partners, parents, siblings, friends, colleagues, business associates, officials, and so on. The list is endless. Relationships are part and parcel of our life, and they can be a sensitive subject for many of us. When you feel that someone whom you thought loved you betrays you and leaves you with what feels to be a broken heart, it's not easy for the ego to forgive and trust others again.

Everyone in life is living their journey on their vibration, and sometimes we need to attract a specific type of energy to help us grow on our path. We may end up in a relationship for many years or just a few months. Still, we tend to stay in that relationship until we have learned the lessons we need to learn to evolve, or otherwise, we will repeat the same experiences with various partners until we learn and change our own conditioned beliefs. This is true of business relationships just as much as personal relationships. You see people making the same mistakes again and again in their business relationships, and this will continue until they have learned from their experiences and changed.

So how does change happen? Change comes with awareness. Once a person moves into a state of present consciousness, then the transformation can begin. You give life to what you focus on. Bringing up pain of a memory or behaviour into your present moment will help you eventually release it, as when the realisation of what has happened or is happening comes into the present state and is accepted. Healing can't happen from a place of illusion, the past or future; that acknowledgment will shift your energy.

Partners and family life

Sometimes other spiritual energies are destined to enter our world and start their life's journey in the form of our children, and for that reason alone, a connection is made with a partner with divine intervention. But that doesn't mean that that relationship was meant to be a long-standing one. The relationship has served its purpose, and the purpose is now over. This was the case with my Sons father and me. The energy of my son was destined to bo born, and for a ohort time, the energy fields of my Sons father and I were on the same wavelength, but very quickly after I fell pregnant that changed. My son was conceived, and his energy was being prepared to enter the world and create its waves. Still, his parent's relationship had to end as those vibrations were creating more chaos and negativity, not harmony. I believe here the Universe had a bigger picture as the combination of my sons' father, and I needed to be manifested through my son for a bigger purpose.

In some situations, a relationship may be unbalanced because one partner is in it for love and the other for different needs, but society has taught us that love is the only respectable pure reason to be in a relationship, yet this is an illusion. What we call love is often perceptions created by us from what we have learned from our own experiences, and from what we've been taught, what we've seen in the media and elsewhere, much of which isn't real, isn't true to life. What we call love, in some people's perspective, could just be a way two people need to behave with each other or things they need to give to each other, simple acts that need to occur, e.g., Moving in together, getting engaged, being married or having children. That's not love it's an illusion of what love is supposed to look like. Being in love and being in a relationship are two very different things. Two people in a relationship may not be in love but are together to satisfy a constructed belief system or for material needs to be met. For this reason, everyone's relationship should be unique and not compared to others. The truth is that both parties are in a relationship to fulfil their needs in some way, whether it be for companionship, children, to ease their insecurities or something more materialistic such as money and status.

Relationships tend to mirror a vibration, a trait or commonality in each person, which is what keeps partners together. When the vibrations of both individuals no longer resonate on the same wavelength, then certain so-called flaws show themselves. It is then that those in the relationship should evaluate what they initially needed from the relationship, what they accept from their partner, and what they were looking for from the relationship and was it fulfilled. Was it themselves that put the pressure on the other person or association to fit the preconceived mould of relationships that they had?

Your relationship with yourself

It is essential to establish a relationship with yourself first. When your relationship with yourself is a strong and unique one with love and respect for yourself, you can then give yourself the time and space to be whole as a human being living your spiritual experience with love. Being complete means expressing every part of yourself as far as possible, so if you have a yearning to paint or be in a choir, then try to do that, because that is part of who you are. Only then will you attract the relationship with your twin soul as both energies will unite as two whole beings and not two separate halves dependent on each other to fill a void. Entering a relationship to fill a void is asking for future failure as anything can happen in life to anyone at any time, and it usually always does. If either party is not prepared, it could only knock everything out of balance.

We need to remind ourselves not to make the pursuit of being in a relationship and find someone to fulfil our needs a constant priority as it can cause intense frustration and desperation within us, which will only detract the relationship that you are looking for. We need to analyse the list of things that we want from a partner and ask ourselves are we giving our self those things. How can we expect those things from someone else if we don't give ourselves those things or, more importantly, if we don't feel we deserve those things? To be whole is to express your masculine and feminine energy, what you expect from a Male, and what you expect from a Female. That doesn't mean you're a feminist, a tomboy, to girly or Alpha; it just means your balanced.

Dealing with rejection

When life's situations take one partner by surprise, and they can't support the other, then it is only to be expected that one partner feels rejected, and they are left with a void which had previously been filled by the other half. It is then that we might turn that rejection into anger towards the other person, but in the long run, that is not the best way forward. Regardless of what has happened in the past, I choose to remain friends even peripherally with some of my ex-partners - at least in the more adult stage of my life! Holding onto any negative feelings regarding my past relationships will only manifest those negative feelings within me and my world, not theirs. It is silly for me to keep harming myself in that way.

Indeed, some of those people have now become my biggest help as my vibration towards them has changed and their vibration towards me also changed. I let go of resistance, fear, intimidation, and more so the others did too. Everything changed and rose to a higher vibration. There is no point in keeping my heart in a negative vibration for anyone from a past relationship. I can only see them as my teachers and guides that helped me recognise things within myself, how I manifested situations in my life, and what I no longer needed in my life. If you harbour negative feelings about a situation that has long gone, those feelings become your current vibration, and that will attract more of the same.

Attracting your soul mate

It is becoming more and more apparent these days that people genuinely want to be with their true love or soul mate. Finding your true love or soul mate can be a meeting of partners that were destined to meet at that time for the growth of the spirit and evolution as a whole. Whether married or living together what matters is that the connection was created from the perspective of a soul journey. The real genuine love connection of two pillows is with a twin soul, and that only comes when we are living in our pure vibration. So, if we wish to meet a particular type of person, we need to make sure our vibration meets theirs. And if we want to keep our relationships in good shape, we need to keep our vibrations high.

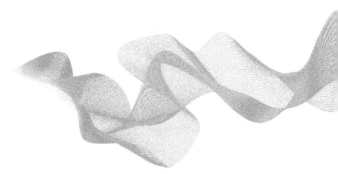

$\mathcal{P}art$ 15

$\mathcal{E}go$ and Compassion

Ego and compassion are like yin and yang. We need both in our lives, but so often, it is ego that dominates. Ego feels the need to be always right regardless of how that may make others feel. Is it necessary to win that point? Is it so important that the ego must win the argument? In any case, how long will you remember that win or that argument? The mind hardly ever remembers, it is quickly gone. Much better to talk with compassion and trust before ego gets carried away. To let the other person win, rather than your ego Is a much stronger action.

I will use the practice of yoga as an example of how ego can lead you to dominate and distort behaviour. When practising yoga, it is important to release any resistance within the body and mind and feel the postures, bringing mind, body, and spirit together. We need to connect and fully embrace yoga with our whole self, inside and out. When that happens, the body and mind will let go of all limiting beliefs and physical tensions, and the body frees itself to raise its vibration to a higher vibration of love. What is the point of doing yoga and showing pictures of ourselves across social media trying to impress the world when, in reality, we may be experiencing pain physically and mentally? That is an example of how ego can take over our behaviour.

Sometimes yoga can challenge us in ways that we may find uncomfortable, and that can discomfort ego too. Yet one of the purposes of yoga is to help us get past obstacles. If you are in an uncomfortable situation, the answer is to find a way to surmount it. However, ego sees an obstacle as a flaw and so may encourage us to ignore it or hate it, whereas if we climb over it, we are no longer uncomfortable, and at the mercy of Ego, we have raised out vibrations. What is true in yoga is also true in life.

Again, in the context of Yoga, sometimes people find an escape in teaching and become a teacher. They can put their perceived problems and the way they see themselves aside, and for a short time, their conditioned reality has changed as their new students look up to them in admiration and respect, and sometimes the teacher needs this to feed their ego. Sometimes a teacher loses themselves in their ego because for them, it is a way to be loved. When students say beautiful things about them, they perceive this as love, but that perception is just massaging their ego. I have always been very wary in my growing years of any Yoga classes I participated in as my spirit would tune into the real essence of the teacher and the teachings of the class. I am the same now with my son and won't let him attend just any Yoga class, I would need to understand the teacher's vibration first. Unfortunately, these days not many Yoga teachers out there teach 'real Yoga.'

Conversely, if a person can walk away from that short-term fix of admiration and respect, that is admirable because it shows that they are willing to be true to themselves and be compassionate towards themselves and others and not try to be something that they're not just to feed their ego.

This is very important to remember as a spiritual teacher because feeding the ego is the very thing that you are supposed to be teaching others not to do. The ego in fact, isn't the problem as it's part of us and will always have to play some role in our lives for us to be the best we can be, but it's when it takes over the compassion that it becomes a problem. The imbalance is the problem. We need ego to function, stand up for ourselves, and to know we are capable of handling anything that comes our way and to know we are the best at what we do. But when we lose ourselves entirely to the ego, then the imbalance will occur.

Many celebrities out there are lost in 'the game of life,' and have become disconnected from their own true power. To be a very big celebrity, the ego must be present, but to sell yourself to fear in exchange for fame and riches simply because you believe you can't have them otherwise, is an illusion. Deep down, your higher self knows you can have anything and be anything that you want to be. It takes complete trust and love in the higher power. Our real self is connected to that higher power; it is much greater than the ego.

The ego grips us when we think it is the route to abundance, but abundance is everywhere and unlimited and can be created as quickly as you visualise it. It manifests as fast as you believe it and know it will. We don't need the mass ego and vibration of fear to help us, because our true nature is fearless. We are love. Unlimited trust in the Universe will bring us all we desire and need and want, but it must be for the good of the Universe. If it is not, then at some point, we may get thrown back to the karmic field of learning and need the help of fear and ego, but this way of behaving can bring many obstacles and difficulties because we are then moving forward with fear and not trust. In any case, the results of this behaviour can be lost as quickly as they appear because the ego needs to be constantly fed with even more energy of fear to supply it with what it needs and what it desires. To get out of the ego's grip is to continually make choices from Love and not fear.

To return to your true self, to love, and to feel compassion is to regain your power. Isn't that where you want to be?

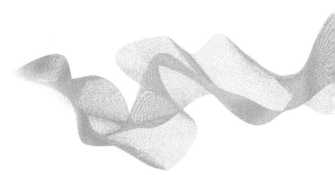

Part 16

The Self

Me, myself, and I. Been through it and seen it all! We can be so protective of our personalities that we forget we are part of something much bigger, part of a whole, and without that whole, we wouldn't be who we are today.

It is so important to recognise that what makes us unique is our truth, and that is our contribution to the whole of life and to the whole of existence. Whatever we decide to do in our life, it is the uniqueness of each one of us that will make it a success - success not only professionally but also in our personal growth and spiritual expansion. Success is an achievement, a perception; that's all it is. It may be seen in other people's eyes as a big or small achievement, but to us, it may be huge! Something that we only dreamed of accomplishing!

It is, therefore, also essential to know yourself and your truth as we all live from our different perspectives and journeys. What we have been through defines who we become. We educate ourselves, we learn and grow, and we evolve as spiritual beings living a human existence. Still, it is important to remember that our life path was chosen by us, ourselves many years ago at birth. It was a path we decided to walk on, to grow as a part of a spiritual family. We need to understand that sometimes there are reasons why things happen to us; it is to learn and evolve from what we experience.

Life is an ocean of learning, so we need not turn our back on any of our experiences but just embrace them all as lessons and evolve. This learning will be sent back to the energy that surrounds our existence, to the matrix that surrounds our planet to benefit the spiritual family on Earth and the growing understanding of consciousness.

We have all gone through heartbreaks and trials, but those things are part of a journey for us to recognise who we are. We go through situations in life to understand what is acceptable to our spirit and to know ourselves entirely from the inside and out. To be untrue and to live a lie when a situation is affecting you or others around you are just prolonging what is happening, and that is not right if you want to be fully present in your life.

To be true from the start may not always seem kind at the time, but it can prevent what could be a testing time later and steer circumstances differently to benefit everyone concerned. We may be faced with this kind of dilemma when we manifest the shadow side of us (the side that we tend to keep hidden within us or choose not to acknowledge for some reason) later in a relationship. Our shadow side can appear as people or situations that take us off guard, and that's when the truth is called for, and we finally find ourselves in the situation with the opportunity to face the shadow side head-on and with strength.

The self is a spiritual being living a human existence, and we need to remember that without the human existence we could never feel the emotions and the heartbreak, experience the learning, and evolve and grow into a higher conscious being. Without the human existence, we could not teach through our own experiences, we could not feel others' and our pain, and nor could we create stunning masterpieces of beautiful music, architecture, art, literature and much more.

Acceptance is to know ourselves, to be present, and to know we have chosen to be here 'to live' come what may. To embrace our learning without resistance is acceptance, and a way to return to the vibration of love, because resistance will only bring more resistance and more pain and suffering. We are here to learn and grow, and when there are people who no longer serve us on our journey in life, we should let them follow whichever path they must walk on so that they can learn and grow. Their way may lead to even more evolving, growing, and spiritual expanding for the vibrational growth of all.

When we are true to ourselves, we let go of resistance to being who we are, and we become open to the higher consciousness. We connect to our inner calling and raise our vibrations to the vibration of Infinite Love. Our vibrational tribe, the love that we seek, the resources that we need, the career that we want, and more will come to us from the higher vibration of love, not the vibration of fear. We can then open our arms to life, not with fear and resistance, but instead with unconditional love and trust, and embrace what the Universe has in store for us. When our vibrations are high, we are on our true path, and it feels like home.

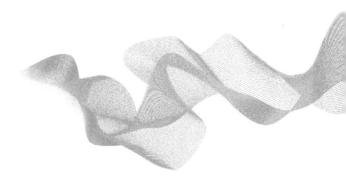

Conclusion

The Vibrational change is already happening on this planet and beyond. To be a higher wavelength helps the individual tune into the changes and understand the new vibrational messages. Children and other highly intelligent beings, including animals, are being born every day already connected to the new vibration and sensitive to the world's toxicity and lower vibrations. They decide to follow a purer, healthier, and more compassionate way of life from a young age. It is up to the adults of the previous generation to allow that evolving process in the growing individual and not to project their fears and insecurity from their day change the evolving spirit.

Raising the vibrations are the only way to protect yourself fully from any negative vibrational energy fields and thought forms bombarding you daily. We, as the public, the general human race on this planet, are not aware of every emitting electromagnetic field, radio wave, radiation, chemical, frequency, and altered food, present in our everyday consumption and interaction. We must accept that there may be things happening that we don't understand and may never comprehend. Still, our protection against these is not to be open, vulnerable, and susceptible to them by remaining on a low vibration.

I was only having a conversation with my son recently, and we were talking about the importance of water and how water itself carries energies and can receive and emit feelings and thought waves. Also, that we are made of around 80% water and communication with each other by repeating a negative word or with a negative thought can only harm the water, alternatively speaking and treating each other respectively can only beautify the water. My son even repeats loving words to water as he showers, now that he has begun to understand the importance and power of the vibrations of water. We must remember for those that live in countries where rain is an abundant element, or should I say where it rains quite often the water itself could be carrying energies, vibrations, and frequencies. Even in the water we drink.

Our protection is to rise above it. Letting go of resistance, the fight, and the vibration of fear, which is a heavy feeling and move up to the vibration of love, a lighter wavelength. One which will no longer leave us defenceless and open to negative energies but rather open the doors to an ocean of unlimited possibilities from a higher perspective and a higher intelligence.

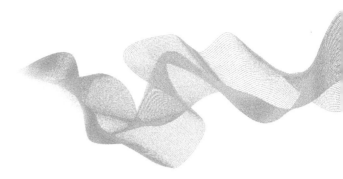

About the Author

Kiran Shashi is a third-generation Yoga teacher with over 20 years' experience and continuing to develop through the discovery of Yoga and spirituality. She holds many certificates from various health systems and organisations which all help to create a foundation for everything she practices and teaches. Her Yoga has earned her a reputation for being unique, compassionate, and defined and become widely recognised in the Health and fitness world as a specialist Yoga teacher.

She has been teaching people and children of all ages and runs yearly retreats and workshops all over the world.

Kiran in Hindi means Light from a candle or Rays from the Sun & Shashi is loosely translated as the ray of moonlight that illuminates our path when in darkness. Like Ying and Yang, combining both provides the perfect symbolic balance of a higher vibration through night and day.

She has been blessed to travel all over the globe with other fitness experts and teach thousands of people, guiding them in fitness and health, including working on more public media platforms.

Her Yoga teachings have gradually widened to running more workshops, courses, writing, and speaking, focused on creating a total wellbeing system for the individual.

This book is the start of her creative expression as a writer and putting her teachings on paper to reach a much wider audience.

After all, not everyone does Yoga!

"I trust this book helps you on your spiritual journey and helps you, not just raise your Vibration but, start the tidal wave of 'A New Vibration,' ready to be experienced by us all!"

Kiran Shashi

Lightning Source UK Ltd.
Milton Keynes UK
UKHW010226280520
363924UK00001BA/108